Multiple Choice
Questions on
Paediatrics

Multiple Choice Questions on Paediatrics

ROY MEADOW
MA BM FRCP DCH DRCOG
Senior Lecturer in Paediatrics and Child Health,
University of Leeds.
Honorary Consultant Paediatrician, Leeds.

BLACKWELL SCIENTIFIC PUBLICATIONS
OXFORD LONDON EDINBURGH MELBOURNE

© 1979 Blackwell Scientific Publications
Osney Mead, Oxford OX2 0EL
8 John Street, London WC1N 2ES
9 Forrest Road, Edinburgh EH1 2QH
P.O. Box 9, North Belwyn, Victoria, Australia

First published 1979

British Library Cataloguing in Publication Data

Meadow, Samuel Roy
    Multiple choice questions on paediatrics
    1. Pediatrics – Problems, exercises, etc.
    I. Title
    618.9′2′00076   RJ48

    ISBN 0–632–00522–X

Distributed in U.S.A. by
Blackwell Mosby Book Distributors
11830 Westline Industrial Drive
St Louis, Missouri 63141,
in Canada by
Blackwell Mosby Book Distributors
86 Northline Road, Toronto
Ontario, M4B 3E5,
and in Australia by
Blackwell Scientific Book Distributors
214 Berkeley Street, Carlton.
Victoria 3053

Set in Monotype Bembo
Printed in Great Britain by Western Printing Services Ltd, Bristol
Bound by Kemp Hall Bindery, Oxford

CONTENTS

PREFACE

Multiple Choice Questions play an important part in most medical examinations, (some of us may feel that they play too large a part). They are a useful method of testing factual knowledge and, in addition, can be helpful as an aid to learning and efficient reading.

I have used these questions with my tutorial groups. The students split up into pairs, discuss the questions, and arrive at an agreed answer before we discuss the answers and the topic as a group. They have found that it is best to be in pairs rather than alone or in a large group; discussion and argument seem to be optimal between two students of similar knowledge.

Whether you use this book on your own or with a partner *do* arrive at an answer of either 'True' 'False' or 'Don't know' before looking up the answers at the back of the book. Commit yourself —for that is the best way to learn. It will also help you to find out how you might improve your scoring in any multiple choice test. It is usual to give for each sub-section a mark of + 1 for a correct answer, − 1 for an incorrect answer and zero for 'Don't know'. The gambler may find he is ruining his chances by too much guessing. The cautious may find that he would do better by backing his hunches and less frequent use of the 'Don't know' option.

The first 150 multiple choice questions are grouped under system headings; the last 25 are mixed for the purpose of revision. The information required to answer these questions should be available in any good paediatric text (including I trust *Lecture Notes on Paediatrics*!). Questions are difficult to construct and I should be grateful for any criticisms, suggestions or alternative answers.

The final section contains some short clinical problems as a relief from multiple choice and to remind the reader that in practice careful attention to the clinical history is the key to correct diagnosis and effective help for the child and family.

Leeds 1979   Roy Meadow

ACKNOWLEDGEMENTS

After complaining in the past about the lengthy gestation period which most publishers require between receiving the completed manuscript and publishing a book, I gratefully acknowledge the speed and efficiency with which Mr Peter Saugman and his colleagues at Blackwell Scientific Publications have produced this book.

I am most grateful to Miss Wendy Haigh and Mrs Aileen Williams for their intelligent and careful assistance.

MULTIPLE CHOICE QUESTIONS

THE NEWBORN AND INFANT FEEDING

1. **Amniocentesis can lead to the prenatal diagnosis of:**
   A severe rhesus haemolytic disease
   B meningomyelocele
   C cystic fibrosis
   D anencephaly
   E hyaline membrane disease

2. **A newborn baby with an Apgar score of 10 should:**
   A be pink all over
   B have a regular respiratory rate above 20 per minute
   C have a heart rate about 70 per minute
   D cry when a catheter is placed in the nostril
   E move all limbs actively

3. **A cephalhaematoma:**
   A is most common over the occipital region
   B does not cross suture lines
   C resolves within 10 days
   D does not require treatment with blood transfusion
   E may exacerbate jaundice in the neonatal period

4. **The main problems of pre-term babies include:**
   A meconium aspiration
   B respiratory distress syndrome
   C hyperbilirubinaemia
   D infections
   E nerve palsy

5. Weakness of the hand muscles is a complication of:
A injury to the upper part of the Brachial plexus (Erb's palsy)
B injury to Auerbach's plexus
C injury to the lower part of the Brachial plexus (Klumpke's palsy)
D injury to the cervical spine
E intraventricular haemorrhage

6. Respiratory distress syndrome is more likely:
A in infants born to mothers who have had corticosteroids during pregnancy
B in infants of diabetic mothers
C to present within the first 12 hours of life than later
D in a 2 kg baby born at 34 weeks gestation than a 1.8 kg baby born at 37 weeks gestation
E to cause permanent lung damage than smoking 20 cigarettes a day during adult life.

7. Characteristic features of physiological jaundice include:
A onset after the first 24 hours of life
B disappearance by the 10th day of life
C a serum bilirubin level below 250 mmol/l
D itching
E associated anaemia

8. Haemorrhagic disease of the newborn:
A is most common in rhesus-positive babies
B is most common about the 2nd or 3rd day of life
C is associated with a prolonged prothrombin time
D is treated with oral Vitamin K
E is commoner in babies who are breast-fed

9. **Mental handicap and eye damage are a well-recognised consequence of prenatal infection with:**
   A cytomegalovirus
   B Epstein–Barr virus
   C rubella virus
   D *Treponema pallidum*
   E *Toxoplasma gondii*

10. **The following statements are true of neonatal convulsions:**
   A hypocalcaemic fits do not cause brain damage
   B they are commoner in low birth weight babies
   C those occurring in the first 2 days have the worst prognosis
   D they are usually followed by seizures later in life
   E anticonvulsant drugs are not indicated

11. **Retrolental fibroplasia is:**
   A primarily a disease of light-for-dates infants
   B a result of disordered development of the retinal blood vessels
   C a result of excessively low $Pa\,O_2$
   D unlikely to cause significant loss of vision
   E more likely in pre-term than post-term infants

12. **The perinatal mortality rate is:**
   A the number of stillbirths and deaths in the first 28 days of life per 1000 total births
   B the number of stillbirths and deaths in the first 7 days of life per 1000 total births
   C about 30% of what it was 30 years ago
   D is in the range of 30–35
   E is lower in the United Kingdom than in any other European country

13. **An infant requires each day:**
    A   45 mg of Vitamin C
    B   110 calories per kg
    C   150 ml of water per kg
    D   400 iu of Vitamin D
    E   6 mg of iron

14. **Human milk differs from cow's milk in the following ways:**
    A   less sodium
    B   more protein
    C   more lactose
    D   more fat
    E   less phosphorus

15. **Breast feeding is considered superior to bottle feeding because:**
    A   iron deficiency anaemia is less likely
    B   most drugs ingested by the mother will be passed on to the baby in the milk
    C   maternal antibody discourages colonisation of the gut by pathogens
    D   bottle-fed babies are psychologically deprived
    E   bottle-fed babies are more prone to gastroenteritis, hypernatraemia and hypocalcaemia

16. **Most modern powdered or liquid milk products for babies:**
    A   have a solute load similar to breast milk
    B   are fortified with Vitamin D, Vitamin C and iron
    C   are derived from cow's milk
    D   are more expensive than whole cow's milk in a bottle
    E   are an inadequate source of food after the age of 2 months

17. **A 4-year-old child who is just below the 3rd percentile for height:**
    A is likely to be unhealthy
    B is approximately 2 standard deviations below the mean normal height for that age
    C is likely to be just below the 3rd percentile for weight
    D is likely to be about the 3rd percentile for height when 2 years older
    E is likely to reach puberty at least a year later than a child who is on the 50th percentile for height

18. **Short stature is associated with:**
    A chronic renal disease
    B malabsorption
    C Down's syndrome
    D emotional deprivation
    E low birth weight

19. **The following groups of children are particularly at risk for rickets:**
    A those aged 5–10 years
    B those from Sikh families living in Britain
    C those from Muslim families living in Britain
    D mentally handicapped children with epilepsy taking long-term phenytoin
    E those with severe renal insufficiency

20. **Important features of nutritional rickets are:**
    A hypertonia
    B raised serum alkaline phosphatase
    C bow legs
    D secondary hyperparathyroidism
    E pica

21. **A British girl aged 13 is likely to have:**
    A   mature breast development (stage 5)
    B   pubic hair extending down the inner surface of the thighs
    C   commenced menstruation
    D   the ability to conceive a child
    E   reached at least 75% of her final adult height

22. **Turner's syndrome is associated with:**
    A   neonatal lymphoedema
    B   a XXX sex chromosome complement
    C   infertility
    D   severe mental handicap
    E   obesity

DEVELOPMENTAL SKILLS

23. **A child aged 8 months is expected:**
    A   to sit without support for 2 minutes
    B   to weigh between 9 and 12 kg
    C   to have a visible molar tooth
    D   to reach out and grasp an object
    E   to turn promptly to sounds made a foot lateral to the ear

24. **A child aged 5 years is expected to:**
    A   copy with a pencil a square shape
    B   have a head circumference within the range 54–56 cm
    C   dress and undress alone
    D   know his name and address
    E   stand on one foot for 5 seconds

25. **A child aged 18 months is expected to:**
   A   build a tower of 3 cubes
   B   pick up a toy from the floor without falling over
   C   show unhappiness when removed from mother
   D   use a spoon competently
   E   be dry by day

26. **A concomitant squint:**
   A   is commoner than a paralytic squint
   B   is considered abnormal only after the age of 6 months
   C   is commonly the result of poor visual acuity
   D   is likely to require surgical correction
   E   may result in permanent amblyopia

27. **A child aged 3 years is expected to:**
   A   copy with a pencil a circle shape
   B   show at least 2 carpal bones on hand X-ray
   C   speak in sentences
   D   walk up and down stairs
   E   be able to hop

28. **Reading backwardness is more common in:**
   A   girls
   B   children from social classes IV and V
   C   Down's syndrome than Turner's syndrome
   D   the children of immigrant families
   E   children born with spina bifida

29. **A child aged 14 months is expected to:**
   A   stand without support for a second or two
   B   wave bye-bye
   C   have a vocabulary of at least 20 words
   D   localise soft sounds made 3 feet above the head
   E   understand simple commands

B

30. **A child of 7 months should have:**
    A an open posterior fontanelle
    B an open anterior fontanelle
    C a symmetrical Moro reflex
    D a brisk response to sounds made $1\frac{1}{2}$ feet lateral to the ear
    E a down-going plantar response (negative Babinski)

31. **Important causes of hypotonia in an infant aged 9 months include:**
    A Down's syndrome
    B cerebral palsy
    C rickets
    D coeliac disease
    E severe mental retardation

32. **The following conditions are generally inherited by sex-linked recessive genes:**
    A Duchenne muscular dystrophy
    B temporal lobe epilepsy
    C meningomyelocele
    D haemophilia
    E Turner's syndrome

33. **Petit mal epilepsy:**
    A may be provoked by hyperventilation
    B does not start before the age of 10
    C is rarely associated with organic brain damage
    D is easily confused with vasovagal attacks
    E is a common sequela of breath-holding attacks

34. **Febrile convulsions usually:**
    A   occur in boys and not girls
    B   occur after the age of 1 year and before the age of 5
    C   last for less than 15 minutes
    D   are associated with upper respiratory tract infection
    E   mean that the child will have epilepsy in later life

35. **Normal cerebrospinal fluid:**
    A   appears clear
    B   has a glucose level similar to the blood glucose level
    C   contains less than 4 lymphocytes/mm³
    D   contains less than 4 polymorphs/mm³
    E   has a protein concentration of 0.4 –1.0 g/litre

36. **The following are common symptoms and signs of meningitis in a school child:**
    A   fever
    B   headache
    C   fits
    D   neck stiffness
    E   palpable occipital glands

37. **The following are important causes of cerebral palsy:**
    A   birth trauma
    B   medulloblastoma
    C   hyperbilirubinaemia
    D   intrauterine infection
    E   non-accidental injury of infants

38. **Spasticity is characterised by, or associated with:**
    A   clonus
    B   quadriplegia
    C   clasp-knife rigidity
    D   persistence of the asymmetric tonic neck reflex
    E   increased tendon reflexes

39. **A sacral meningomyelocele is commonly associated with:**
   A   spasticity of the lower legs
   B   hydrocephalus
   C   a neuropathic bladder
   D   multiple haemangiomata
   E   a lax anal sphincter

40. **Important symptoms or signs of a space-occupying lesion are:**
   A   headache
   B   visual disturbances
   C   neck stiffness
   D   earache
   E   a raised CSF protein

MENTAL HANDICAP

41. **The following conditions cause mental handicap:**
   A   nephrogenic diabetes insipidus
   B   galactosaemia
   C   hypothyroidism
   D   tuberose sclerosis
   E   cystinosis

42. **Children attending classes for the moderately educationally subnormal (ESNM):**
   A   are more numerous than those in classes for severely educationally subnormal (ESNS)
   B   are likely to have an intelligence quotient of less than 50
   C   are unlikely to be able to fend for themselves in later life
   D   commonly have other congenital abnormalities
   E   are most likely to come from a family of lower social class and low intelligence

43. **A mongol girl:**
   A has 49 chromosomes
   B is likely to have a first degree relative who is also a mongol
   C is more likely to result from the union of a 37-year-old mother and a 30-year-old father, than from a 30-year-old mother and a 40-year-old father
   D shows Barr bodies in the buccal smear
   E is usually the result of chromosome non-disjunction

44. **A mongol boy is likely to grow up into a man who:**
   A has children half of whom will be mongols
   B has an intelligence quotient of less than 50
   C has a life expectancy less than a man with cystic fibrosis
   D is below average height
   E has recurrent seizures

45. **The head circumference:**
   A should be measured round the occipito-frontal perimeter
   B is larger in boys than in girls
   C is normally related to body size
   D is irrelevant after the age of 5
   E is normal in craniostenosis

46. **The following are common features of Down's syndrome:**
   A hypotonia
   B a small head circumference
   C clinodactyly
   D recurrent respiratory tract infections
   E pigmented birth marks

47. **Features of periodic syndrome include:**
    A   a mode age below the age of 5
    B   an abnormal EEG
    C   unilateral abdominal pain
    D   low intelligence
    E   vomiting

48. **Children with nocturnal enuresis:**
    A   account for 10–15% of 5-year-olds
    B   commonly have a first degree relative who also had nocturnal enuresis
    C   are generally slow to acquire other skills also
    D   should not be treated with drugs below the age of 5
    E   usually have frequency of micturition by day

49. **Tics (habit spasms):**
    A   are more common in girls than in boys
    B   most commonly involve the hands
    C   are best treated with antidepressant drugs
    D   are an indication for referral to a Child Guidance Clinic
    E   generally recur for at least 6 months

50. **Faecal soiling is:**
    A   commonly associated with meningomyelocele
    B   a frequent result of severe constipation
    C   abnormal after the age of 5
    D   an indication for rectal examination
    E   the presenting feature of Hirschsprung's disease

51. Nightmares:

A are common
B are a sign of severe emotional disturbance
C occur during non-REM sleep
D cannot be remembered on waking up
E are precipitated by hypnotic drugs

52. Breath-holding attacks:

A are commoner over the age of $3\frac{1}{2}$ years
B are easily confused with a generalised seizure
C may be precipitated by a minor injury
D should be treated with sedatives
E are an important cause of brain damage

53. The following are important features of infantile autism:

A slowness in learning to talk
B failure to make warm emotional relationships
C slow development of gross motor skills
D infantile 'spasms'
E constipation

54. The following are common features of childhood migraine

A associated travel sickness
B a family history of migraine
C unilateral headache
D a headache lasting less than 2 minutes
E provocation by chocolate or cheese

55. **The following are usually associated with severe psychological disturbance:**
   A   masturbation in a pre-school child
   B   nightmares in an adolescent
   C   thumb sucking in a school child
   D   temper tantrums in a toddler
   E   head banging in an infant

CARDIOVASCULAR SYSTEM

56. **The following are likely to be normal in a 5-year-old child:**
   A   a blood pressure of 135/90
   B   a palpable systolic thrill
   C   a third heart sound
   D   a split second heart sound
   E   a pulse rate of 100 per minute

57. **The blood pressure is likely to appear higher if:**
   A   the child is standing
   B   the child is crying
   C   too large a sphygmomanometer cuff is used
   D   the flush method of determination is used
   E   the child is receiving corticosteroid therapy

58. **Cardiac failure in infancy is characterised by:**
   A   a respiratory rate of more than 40 per minute
   B   a heart rate of more than 150 per minute
   C   absent femoral pulses
   D   enlarged palpable liver
   E   feeding difficulty

59. **There is an increased incidence of heart disease in:**
    A people who have had rheumatic fever
    B children who have had rubella
    C mongols
    D Turner's syndrome
    E children with diabetes mellitus

60. **A ventricular-septal defect:**
    A usually causes cardiac failure in infancy
    B is associated with a pan-systolic murmur
    C is associated with plaeonaemic lung fields on chest X-ray
    D may close spontaneously as the child becomes older
    E is usually associated with a conduction defect

61. **Patent ductus arteriosus:**
    A is a left-to-right shunt
    B is associated with a high volume peripheral pulse
    C generally requires surgical correction
    D tends to cause clubbing of the fingers
    E is associated with a characteristic murmur best heard at the back

62. **Hypertension in a girl:**
    A may be cause by atrial septal defect
    B is commoner than in a boy
    C may be the result of renal disease
    D is most likely to be 'essential' hypertension
    E is more likely if the parents are hypertensive

63. **Fallot's tetralogy is associated with:**
    A oligaemic lung fields on chest X-ray
    B death by the age of 3 years unless corrected by surgery
    C a widely split second heart sound
    D a raised systolic blood pressure
    E central cyanosis

64. Children aged 4:
A commonly develop otitis media
B commonly have sinusitis
C are too young to be tested by audiometry
D are too young to wear a hearing aid
E commonly have palpable cervical lymph glands

65. The following are features of acute otitis media:
A discharge from the ear
B pain in the ear
C buzzing in the ear
D a red eardrum
E neck stiffness

66. Indications for tonsillectomy are:
A recurrent colds
B recurrent wheezy bronchitis
C recurrent bouts of acute tonsillitis
D adenoidectomy
E otitis media

67. Stridor in a 2-year-old:
A may be normal
B is best heard on expiration
C may be the result of *Haemophilus influenzae* infection
D rarely lasts longer than 3 days
E may be caused by an inhaled foreign body

68. **Bronchiolitis is commonly associated with:**
    A measles
    B respiratory syncytial virus
    C onset in winter
    D an age of under 12 months
    E a respiratory rate of over 40 per minute

69. **The following are commonly associated with childhood asthma:**
    A a raised serum IgE level
    B a family history of enuresis
    C a positive skin test to house dust mite
    D a previous history of infantile eczema
    E wheezing after exercise

70. **The following are useful for the treatment of status asthmaticus:**
    A intravenous diazepam
    B intravenous adrenalin
    C disodiumcromoglycate by inhalation
    D intravenous aminophylline
    E intravenous hydrocortisone

71. **Lobar pneumonia:**
    A is commoner in children under the age of 4 than in school children
    B is usually caused by *Strep. pneumoniae*
    C is commonly caused by *Staph. pyogenes*
    D often gives rise to a pleural rub
    E generally causes the child to be ill for over 2 weeks

72. **Staphylococcal pneumonia:**
   A   is common in childhood
   B   is a common complication of cystic fibrosis
   C   is characterised by lung abscesses on X-ray
   D   is best treated with ampicillin
   E   presents with stridor

ALIMENTARY TRACT

73. **The following are likely to be normal in an infant of 3 months:**
   A   a liver palpable 2 cm below the right costal margin
   B   a spleen palpable 1 cm below the left costal margin
   C   a palpable right kidney
   D   undescended testicles
   E   no teeth apparent

74. **Polyhydramnios is associated with:**
   A   renal agenesis
   B   oesophageal atresia
   C   rectal atresia
   D   congenital club foot
   E   anencephaly

75. **In infancy inguinal herniae:**
   A   are commoner in boys
   B   require prompt surgical correction even when they are reducible
   C   do not strangulate in girls
   D   are usually associated with umbilical herniae
   E   are a feature of many syndromes involving multiple congenital abnormalities

76. **Features of infantile pyloric stenosis include:**
   A vomiting of progressive severity
   B anorexia
   C loose motions
   D onset within the first 21 days of life
   E absence of mucus in the vomit

77. **Children with gastroenteritis:**
   A usually yield a pathogenic *E. coli* in their stools
   B require treatment with an antibiotic which is not absorbed from the gut
   C may have blood in their stools
   D do not become severely dehydrated after the age of 4 years
   E often have severe abdominal pain

78. **A child with gluten enteropathy:**
   A generally presents before the age of 2 months
   B shows sub-total villous atrophy on jejunal biopsy
   C has a faecal fat content of less than 3 grams per day
   D has anorexia
   E can usually tolerate rye but not wheat

79. **Important features of herpetic stomatitis include:**
   A vesicles and ulcers on the buccal mucosa as well as the tongue and palate
   B inflamed gums
   C pain
   D recent contact with chicken pox
   E cervical lymph gland enlargement

80. **Blood-stained stools in an infant are associated with:**
    A severe constipation
    B gastroenteritis
    C nose bleeds
    D intussusception
    E coeliac disease

81. **The following are common features of cystic fibrosis:**
    A autosomal recessive inheritance
    B presentation with intestinal obstruction in the newborn
    C offensive stools as a toddler
    D umbilical hernia in infancy
    E staphylococcal pneumonia in the school child

82. **Threadworms:**
    A are common in school children
    B cause diarrhoea
    C cause bedwetting
    D cause abdominal pain
    E cause eosinophilia

83. **The following investigations are particularly useful in the diagnosis of cystic fibrosis:**
    A chest X-ray
    B ECG
    C full blood count
    D sweat sodium concentration
    E barium meal X-ray

SKELETAL SYSTEM AND CONNECTIVE TISSUE DISORDERS

84. **Congenital dislocation of the hip:**
   A   usually requires correction by operative surgery before the age of 2 years
   B   is commoner in girls
   C   is commoner in children with spina bifida
   D   may cause apparent shortening of one leg
   E   is commoner in pre-term babies than those born at 40 weeks gestation

85. **A schoolboy who presents with a 3-day illness caused by acute osteomyelitis is likely to have:**
   A   severe localised pain
   B   fever
   C   neutrophil leucocytosis
   D   an abnormal limb X-ray
   E   a blood culture growth of staphylococci

86. **Permanent joint damage may result from:**
   A   Henoch–Schönlein syndrome
   B   rheumatic fever
   C   tuberculosis
   D   Still's disease
   E   haemophilia

87. **Pathognomonic rashes of rheumatic fever include:**
   A   purpura on lateral aspects of the buttocks
   B   erythema nodosum on the back
   C   erythema marginatum on the trunk
   D   erythema multiforme of the limbs
   E   papular urticaria on the legs

88. **A child with rheumatic fever is likely to:**
   A show choreiform movements of the upper limbs
   B have had lobar pneumonia 2–6 weeks previously
   C show a sustained rise of the anti-streptolysin O titre
   D have a systolic cardiac murmur
   E be over the age of 6 years

89. **Henoch–Schönlein syndrome is associated with:**
   A thrombocytopenic purpura
   B mitral stenosis
   C glomerulonephritis
   D characteristic lesions in the mouth
   E abdominal pain

THE SKIN

90. **The following birth marks usually fade and disappear by adult life:**
   A Mongolian blue spot
   B strawberry naevus
   C port-wine stain
   D pigmented mole
   E stork mark

91. **Features of childhood eczema include:**
   A itching
   B involvement of extensor surfaces by school age
   C a family history suggesting atopy
   D onset before the age of 12 months
   E lymphadenopathy

92. **Important causes of erythema nodosum include:**
   A   tuberculosis
   B   sulphonamide administration
   C   Henoch–Schönlein syndrome
   D   streptococcal infection
   E   congenital heart disease

93. **A Mongolian blue spot is common in:**
   A   Indians
   B   West-Indians
   C   Down's syndrome
   D   the lumbo-sacral region
   E   Chinese children

94. **The following conditions often have a strong genetic predisposition:**
   A   eczema
   B   impetigo
   C   psoriasis
   D   erythema nodosum
   E   scabies

URINARY TRACT

95. **The fetus in the womb:**
   A   has a serum urea greater than 10 mmol/l
   B   does not pass urine until the third trimester of pregnancy
   C   may be associated with oligohydramnios if there is renal agenesis
   D   will be stillborn if there is only one kidney
   E   has produced the total number of nephrons by full term

96. **Cloudy urine is associated with the following substances in the urine:**
    A chemical deposits
    B bacteria
    C blood
    D albumin
    E colouring from candy-floss

97. **The following findings on microscopy of a fresh early morning midstream urine specimen from a boy of 8 are abnormal:**
    A a white cell count of 50 per mm^3
    B a red cell count of 10 per mm^3
    C a granular cast
    D a hyaline cast
    E motile bacteria

98. **The following conditions are inherited by Mendelian patterns of inheritance:**
    A polycystic disease
    B nephrogenic diabetes insipidus
    C posterior urethral valve
    D 'minimal change' nephrotic syndrome
    E Henoch–Schönlein nephritis

99. **The following findings in fresh urine require further investigation:**
    A an albumin concentration of 0.6 g/l
    B a positive reaction for haemoglobin
    C an ammoniacal smell
    D a pH of 5
    E ketonuria

100. **Circumcision is usually required for the following boys:**
   A Jewish, after the age of 4 weeks
   B Sikh
   C West-Indian
   D Muslim
   E Hindu

101. **The urine of a child with nephrotic syndrome is likely to:**
   A be frothy
   B be of small volume
   C show a highly selective differential protein clearance pattern
   D contain excess white cells
   E reveal microscopic haematuria

102. **Post-streptococcal glomerulonephritis characteristically:**
   A occurs in pre-school children
   B follows one or two weeks after a *Strep. pneumonia* infection
   C is associated with generalised oedema
   D requires confinement to bed for at least 4 weeks
   E is a rare cause of end-stage renal failure

103. **Nephrotic syndrome is characterised by:**
   A hypertension
   B heavy proteinuria
   C hypoalbuminaemia
   D reduced serum complement
   E raised blood urea

104. **Urinary tract infection:**
    A   is commoner in girls
    B   is commonly caused by *E. coli*
    C   should be treated by a course of antibiotics lasting at least 4 weeks
    D   is associated with vesico-ureteric reflux
    E   is diagnosed by a colony count of more than 10^6 organisms/l

105. **Routine management of a boy with urinary tract infection would include:**
    A   avoidance of bubble baths
    B   encouragement to void frequently
    C   a kidney X-ray
    D   a course of chemotherapy
    E   measurement of the blood urea

106. **The following features are likely to be seen in a child of 3 with chronic renal insufficiency originating from dysplastic kidneys:**
    A   a haemoglobin of less than 8 g/dl
    B   short stature
    C   oliguria
    D   bow legs
    E   hypertension

HAEMATOLOGY AND ONCOLOGY

107. **The following haematological findings would be considered normal in a 3-month-old infant:**
    A   haemoglobin concentration of 11.5 g/dl
    B   a white cell count of 12.0 × 10^9/l
    C   more lymphocytes than neutrophil polymorphs
    D   an eosinophil count of 0.61 × 10^9/l
    E   a 10% concentration of HbF

108. **The following conditions are commonly controlled by sex-linked recessive genes:**
   A thalassaemia
   B haemophilia A
   C haemophilia B
   D glucose-6-phosphate dehydrogenase deficiency
   E hereditary spherocytosis

109. **Iron deficiency anaemia is associated with:**
   A a low mean corpuscular volume (MCV)
   B raised serum ferritin
   C a mean corpuscular haemoglobin concentration of less than 32 g/dl
   D acanthocytosis
   E a reticulocyte count of less than 5%

110. **Children from Pakistan living in Britain are more likely to develop the following conditions than children of European origin:**
   A Sickle cell disease
   B thalassaemia
   C glucose-6-phosphate dehydrogenase deficiency
   D iron deficiency anaemia
   E pernicious anaemia

111. **The following foods are important sources of iron in childhood:**
   A eggs
   B bread
   C proprietary brands of powdered cow's milk
   D potatoes
   E green vegetables

112. **Characteristic symptoms and signs of sickle-cell disease include:**
    A   acute abdominal pain
    B   acute limb pain
    C   disseminated intravascular thromboses
    D   leucocytosis
    E   fever

113. **Splenomegaly is a feature of:**
    A   haemolytic anaemia
    B   folic acid deficiency anaemia
    C   septicaemia
    D   acute lymphoblastic leukaemia
    E   haemophilia

114. **The following conditions are associated with thrombocytopenic purpura:**
    A   scurvy
    B   Henoch–Schönlein syndrome
    C   leukaemia
    D   severe renal insufficiency
    E   meningococcal septicaemia

115. **A nephroblastoma (Wilm's tumour) is likely to present:**
    A   before the age of 4 years
    B   with abdominal pain
    C   with an enlarged abdomen
    D   with visible abnormality of the urine
    E   with hypertension

116. **The following statements are true of malignant disease in childhood:**
   A   it is the commonest cause of death in school children
   B   permanent cure does not occur
   C   tumours of the nervous system are the commonest form of malignancy
   D   it is not inherited
   E   new cases are twice as common as they were 20 years ago

METABOLIC DISORDERS

117. **Congenital hypothyroidism (cretinism) is characterised by:**
   A   prolonged neonatal jaundice
   B   single palmar creases
   C   feeding difficulty in infancy
   D   a shrill 'cerebral' cry
   E   hypotonia

118. **Adrenogenital syndrome is associated with:**
   A   sex-linked inheritance
   B   over-production of ACTH
   C   vomiting in the neonatal period
   D   undescended testicles
   E   convulsions in the neonatal period

119. **Diabetes mellitus in childhood:**
   A   requires treatment with insulin
   B   occurs most commonly in obese children
   C   is an important cause of childhood renal failure
   D   may resolve as adulthood is reached
   E   is commoner than it was 30 years ago

120. **The following are useful for the diagnosis of cretinism:**
    A serum cholesterol level
    B X-ray of the knees
    C measurement of the head circumference
    D measurement of the neck circumference
    E plasma thyroxine level

121. **The following conditions are causes of permanent mental handicap:**
    A adrenogenital syndrome
    B galactosaemia
    C Cushing's syndrome
    D phenylketonuria
    E hypoglycaemia

122. **The following would be expected in a child with nephrogenic diabetes insipidus:**
    A urine osmolality of less than 400
    B male sex
    C craving for salt
    D antidiuretic hormone deficiency
    E failure to thrive in infancy and growth retardation

123. **The Guthrie test:**
    A must be done on a fresh specimen of urine
    B depends upon the inhibition of bacterial growth by phenylalanine
    C should be done within the first 48 hours of life
    D is unreliable if the baby has jaundice
    E is a radio-immunoassay

THERAPEUTICS

124. **Well-recognised methods of reducing a high fever include:**
   A taking a cold bath
   B oral paracetamol
   C salicylate rectal suppository
   D oral barbiturates
   E removal of clothes

125. **A special diet is usually advised for children with:**
   A hypothyroidism
   B a blood urea higher than 12 mmol/l
   C diabetes mellitus
   D hypertension
   E galactosaemia

126. **Games and PE at school are not advised for children with:**
   A epilepsy
   B periodic syndrome
   C recurrent respiratory tract infections
   D nephrotic syndrome
   E hydrocephalus

127. **Swimming is not advisable for a child who has:**
   A epilepsy
   B eczema
   C chronic otitis media
   D asthma
   E recurrent urinary tract infection

128. **Prolonged phenytoin therapy is associated with:**
 A coarsening of the facial features
 B rickets
 C gum hyperplasia
 D hirsutism
 E intellectual deterioration

129. **Well-recognised complications of corticosteroid therapy include:**
 A glycosuria
 B precocious puberty
 C stunting of height
 D raised blood pressure
 E tinnitus

IMMUNISATION AND INFECTIOUS DISEASES

130. **The following substances cross the placenta freely:**
 A immunoglobulin G
 B immunoglobulin M
 C pethidine
 D urea
 E corticosteroids

131. **By the age of 3 years a child living in Britain should have been immunised against:**
 A tuberculosis
 B poliomyelitis
 C diphtheria
 D mumps
 E tetanus

132. The following immunisations are generally performed using a live organism:
A poliomyelitis
B measles
C rubella
D smallpox
E whooping cough

133. Pertussis vaccine should not be given:
A to a child under the age of 6 months
B to a child with cerebral palsy
C orally
D to a child who has had fits
E At the same time as another immunisation procedure

134. Rubella vaccine:
A is given by intramuscular injection
B is given to all children between the ages of 11 and 14
C should not be given to pregnant women
D should not be given to anyone thought to have had rubella
E provides immunity for a maximum of 4 years

135. BCG
A is given subcutaneously
B is given intradermally
C commonly causes enlarged painful axillary glands
D commonly causes local induration for more than 2 months
E is required by over 90% of British school children over the age of 10

136. **Features of mumps in childhood include:**
    A   an incubation period of around 18 days
    B   parotitis
    C   orchitis
    D   meningitis
    E   lymphopenia

137. **Features of whooping cough in infancy include:**
    A   an incubation period of around 10 days
    B   Koplik's spots
    C   a paroxysmal cough
    D   pneumonia
    E   lymphopenia

138. **The following infections may be caused by farmyard animals:**
    A   glandular fever
    B   tuberculosis
    C   poliomyelitis
    D   brucellosis
    E   chicken pox

139. **A child presenting with tuberculous meningitis:**
    A   is likely to have been ill for at least 2 weeks
    B   should be notified to the Area Environmental Health Officer
    C   may incur permanent brain damage
    D   will have raised levels of protein and white cells in the CSF
    E   will have a normal chest X-ray

140. **Glandular fever is associated with:**
    A histoplasmosis
    B Epstein–Barr virus
    C a polymorphonuclearleucocytosis
    D splenomegaly
    E pancreatitis

141. **A child presenting with the rash of measles will generally have:**
    A fever, cough and conjunctivitis
    B a rash on the face
    C a rash on the hands
    D a raised measles antibody titre
    E eosinophilia

142. **Congenital rubella is associated with:**
    A raised IGM level in the neonate
    B perceptive deafness
    C cataract
    D Down's syndrome
    E neonatal jaundice

143. **Vaccination against smallpox is not recommended for:**
    A anyone with eczema
    B most British children
    C clinical doctors
    D anyone who has had chicken pox
    E pregnant women

ACCIDENTS

144. The following statements apply to accidental poisoning in childhood:
A it is commoner in the pre-school child than the school child
B drugs are a commoner cause of morbidity and mortality than household and garden products
C berries and seeds rarely cause serious illness in the British Isles
D activated charcoal given orally is useful general therapy
E desferrioxamine is useful specific therapy for salicylate poisoning

145. Pharmacologically induced emesis or gastric lavage are contraindicated in the following circumstances:
A if the poison has been ingested more than 3 hours earlier
B ingestion of caustic soda
C ingestion of a piece of chalk
D ingestion of paraffin
E if the child is below the age of 2

146. Chronic lead poisoning is associated with:
A pica
B abdominal pain
C anaemia
D abnormal bone X-ray
E diarrhoea

147. **Accidents are an important cause of morbidity in childhood and:**
   A are the commonest cause of death in school children
   B deaths from poisoning are more common than from non-accidental injury (battered baby syndrome)
   C deaths from burns are more common than deaths from drowning
   D road accidents are the commonest cause of death
   E are commoner in girls than in boys

148. **The following are features of non-accidental injury (battered baby syndrome):**
   A a mode age of 18–24 months
   B multiple fractures of the ribs
   C sub-periosteal haematoma of the long bones
   D sub-hyaloid haemorrhage
   E sub-dural haematoma

149. **Cot deaths are more common in:**
   A males
   B social class V
   C infants over the age of 6 months
   D infants of low birth weight
   E the winter

150. **Death from road accidents would be less if:**
   A children were forbidden to travel in the front seat of the car
   B children were forbidden to read in the car
   C children were made to wear safety belts
   D carry-cots for infants were strapped to the back seat of the car rather than left loose
   E it was forbidden to ride a motor cycle until the age of 18

MISCELLANEOUS

151. Girls of Pakistani parents are:
A likely to be Muslim (the Islam religion)
B at risk for thalassaemia major
C at risk for sickle-cell disease
D given the title Kaur as one of their names
E likely to avoid eating pork

152. Illegitimate babies:
A are usually adopted
B have a greater chance of being born to a mother under the age of 20 than an offspring born in wedlock
C comprise about 9% of all live births
D are associated with an increased perinatal mortality rate
E are placed under a Supervision Order at birth

153. Vesico-ureteric reflux:
A is found in about 25% of schoolgirls with 'asymptomatic' bacteriuria
B requires surgical correction by the age of 8 years
C may be associated with kidney damage
D is identified by an intravenous pyelogram
E is an important cause of nocturnal enuresis

154. A boy need not attend school if he is:
A under the age of 5 years
B over the age of 15 years
C over the age of 15 years and has a paid job which occupies at least two hours each day
D classified as suffering from severe visual impairment
E subject to a 'Supervision Order'

155. Antibiotics are an important part of the treatment of:
   A   bronchiolitis
   B   impetigo
   C   otitis media
   D   acute glomerulonephritis
   E   gastroenteritis

156. A child who is the subject of a Care Order is likely:
   A   to be supervised by the Probation Department
   B   to have only one living parent
   C   to have a severe medical disorder
   D   to have parental rights transferred to the local authority
   E   to have regular contact with a social worker

157. A positive Tuberculin test:
   A   is associated with previous BCG immunisation
   B   may be absent in severe tuberculous meningitis
   C   does not occur after the age of 1 year
   D   should be elicited by subcutaneous injection of Tuber-
        culin
   E   is characterised by induration present 2 days after the
        test

158. Vomiting in infancy is a feature of:
   A   Hirschsprung's disease
   B   pyloric stenosis
   C   hiatus hernia
   D   adreno-genital syndrome
   E   light-for-dates babies

159. **Children with the following features cannot be adopted:**
   A Age over 5 years
   B Hydrocephalus
   C A Roman Catholic mother
   D A congenital heart lesion
   E Natural parents of different colour

160. **The stools of breast-fed babies tend to differ from bottle-fed babies in the following ways:**
   A more frequent
   B more loose
   C more odour
   D more brown
   E more undigested fat

161. **Important consequences of rheumatic fever in later life include:**
   A ankylosing spondylitis
   B mitral stenosis
   C coarctation of the aorta
   D choreoathetoid cerebral palsy
   E renal insufficiency

162. **The following statements are approximately true:**
   A one pound weight = 450 grams
   B 1000 millilitres = 1 litre
   C 20 fluid ounces = 1 pint
   D one litre = 1.76 pints
   E one inch = 0.0254 metre

163. **The following are indications for circumcision:**
   A   hypospadias
   B   a long foreskin
   C   recurrent balanitis
   D   non-retractile foreskin at age of 2 years
   E   if the father has had cancer of the penis

164. **Considering the incidence of the conditions it can be expected that a general practitioner will encounter more children presenting with:**
   A   respiratory tract infection than urinary tract infection
   B   seizures than diabetes mellitus
   C   muscular dystrophy than cerebral palsy
   D   mental handicap than congenital dislocation of the hip
   E   spina bifida than phenylketonuria

165. **Fallot's tetralogy is made up of:**
   A   right ventricular hypertrophy
   B   pulmonary artery arising from left ventricle
   C   over-riding aorta
   D   pulmonary stenosis
   E   ventricular septal defect

166. **Boys of Hindu parents:**
   A   are frequently brought up as vegetarians
   B   are given the title Singh as one of their names
   C   are likely to avoid eating beef
   D   are usually circumcised
   E   frequently have a Mongolian blue spot on their back

167. **The following disorders are commoner in the children of parents of social class V than social class I:**
   A accidents and poisoning
   B malignant disease
   C major congenital abnormalities
   D measles
   E asthma

168. **Acute laryngotracheitis:**
   A occurs most commonly in the child under the age of 4 years
   B generally follows a 3/4 day prodromal illness
   C presents with stridor
   D usually results from bacterial infection
   E can cause severe respiratory distress and obstruction

169. **A neonate with Trisomy 21 is more likely to have the following features than a normal neonate:**
   A a third fontanelle
   B a cardiac murmur
   C hyperbilirubinaemia
   D hyaline-membrane disease
   E intestinal obstruction

170. **Concerning the causes of death in childhood during the last 40 years, it is true to say now that:**
   A death from neoplasm is twice as common
   B death from accidents is twice as common
   C death from infection is at least 10 times less common
   D death in the first month of life is at least two times less common
   E death from diabetes mellitus is more common

171. A 14-year-old boy who has recently returned from a four week holiday with grandparents in Pakistan is at risk of developing:
A smallpox
B malaria
C kwashiorkor
D rickets
E tuberculosis

172. Breathlessness on feeding is a feature of an infant with:
A pyloric stenosis
B cardiac failure
C respiratory tract infection
D tracheo-oesophageal fistula
E mental handicap

173. The following sugars are disaccharides:
A galactose
B fructose
C lactose
D maltose
E sucrose

174. Radiological evidence of chronic pyelonephritis includes:
A cortical scarring
B nephrocalcinosis
C hydronephrosis
D clubbing of the calyces
E kidneys of different size

175. **The following conditions are usually associated with characteristic skin disorders:**
   A galactosaemia
   B Sturge–Weber syndrome
   C Henoch–Schönlein syndrome
   D diabetes mellitus
   E tuberose sclerosis

CASE STUDIES

CASE 1

A 4-week-old boy is admitted to hospital because of vomiting. He is the second child of healthy West-Indian parents. He was born at the end of a normal pregnancy and weighed 3.4 kg. He was breast fed for one week until his mother changed to bottle feeding. At that stage he began to vomit after and between feeds. For the previous two days the vomit contained slime and, on one occasion, blood. For the previous two weeks he had opened his bowels less than once a day.

On examination he is a thin, pale, drowsy baby weighing 3.6 kg. He is floppy and has an umbilical hernia of 2.5 cm diameter. The head circumference is 38 cm with an anterior fontanelle 3 cm in diameter and sunken. Blood tests reveal: haemoglobin 18 g/dl; WBC 15 × 10⁹/l; plasma urea 15 mmol/l. The urine appears dark, is of pH 6, strongly positive for ketones, and has a trace of albumin.

a What therapeutic manoeuvre is required?
b What diagnostic manoeuvre is required?
c What is the best management of the umbilical hernia?

CASE 2

A 3-year-old girl has recurrent attacks which are described by the mother as follows: 'She suddenly gasps, stops breathing, goes red in the face then blue, then falls unconscious to the ground. Sometimes she twitches when unconscious and once she wet herself. The first one came on after she had banged her head on the table, the second when crying after I had told her she couldn't go outside. They are now happening as often as twice a day and last for at least a minute. She seems all right afterwards.'

a What are these attacks?
b What causes them?
c What is the prognosis?
d Is drug therapy indicated?

CASE 3

A baby of 5 months has recurrent episodes 'when he suddenly jumps and throws out his arms and nods his head forward'. He is otherwise healthy.

On examination he looks normal, the skull circumference is 40 cm and his developmental skills are in the range 3–5 months. The perinatal history was normal and the family history is also normal.

a What is the differential diagnosis?
b What special investigation is indicated and in what way might it be abnormal?
c What is the prognosis?

CASE 4

A boy aged 4 years is noticed by his parents to have a swollen face. His urine is frothy in the toilet. He is a bit bad tempered but does not seem ill despite the fact that he is 'just recovering from a cold'. On examination there is generalised oedema and mild ascites, the blood pressure, pulse rate and heart sounds are normal. He has had no serious previous illnesses. His father had epilepsy and there are two healthy siblings.

a What is the probable diagnosis?
b What two confirmatory investigations are required?
c What is the prognosis?
d What drug is likely to be required?

CASE 5

A 4-year-old boy became ill while staying at the family holiday cottage in Scotland. He had a 'runny nose' during the day and then at 11.00 p.m. awoke breathless and crying. He had had two similar but milder episodes, one the previous year when in the holiday cottage, and the other after a cousin's birthday party.

On examination his height is 97 cm and weight 16 kg. There is respiratory distress with flaring of the alar nasae and indrawing of the subcostal region. The respiratory rate is 44 per minute, pulse rate 100 per minute. Generalised rhonchi, most marked on expiration, can be heard.

a Which two conditions would you put at the top of your list of differential diagnoses?
b In which aspects of the family history are you most interested?
c Give at least two explanations for the way in which the circumstances and location of the attacks might be relevant?

CASE 6

A 3-year-old presents with a fever and sore mouth. For 2 days she has refused to eat and has been very miserable. On examination there are many small ulcers on the inside of her mouth. Her gums are involved also, are a dusky red, and bleeding a little. The cervical glands are enlarged and tender. Otherwise she seems healthy and in particular she has no rash on the rest of her body. Apart from a severe respiratory infection (probably bronchiolitis) at the age of 9 months she has been healthy.

a What is the diagnosis?
b What is the cause?
c What is the chance of recurrence?

CASE 7

A 1½-year-old Cypriot child presents with poor weight gain, irritability, and feeding difficulty. He is pale. Developmental assessment suggests that he behaves more like a one-year-old than a 1½-year-old.

The blood picture is as follows: Hb 8.0 g/dl; MCV 70 u³; MCHC 30%; WBC 10 × 10⁹/l; (neutrophils 30%; lymphocytes 60%); ESR 20.

a What type of anaemia is present?
b What is the likely reason for it?
c In view of the poor developmental skills what other aspects of the history is of particular importance?
d Why is the absence of splenomegaly of particular importance?

CASE 8

A 3-year-old boy is admitted to hospital because of a severe pneumonia. Physical examination reveals a rather underweight boy who is febrile and has signs of a right pleural effusion. Chest X-ray appears to show an abscess cavity in the right upper zone. It is the fourth severe respiratory tract infection that the boy has had.

He is the only child of healthy parents. The pregnancy was normal, but during the neonatal period he had prolonged jaundice and severe constipation.

a What is the most likely cause of the pneumonia?
b Suggest an underlying cause and two useful confirmatory symptoms or investigations?

CASE 9

A 22-year-old Indian mother is delivered of a 2 kg baby by breech delivery at the end of a 39 week pregnancy. The early pregnancy was spent in India, and was complicated by considerable vomiting and an 'influenza like' illness about the third month.

After delivery the baby had an Apgar score of 6 at one minute and 10 at four minutes. She appeared healthy but small. On the second day jaundice became apparent and by the fourth day her serum bilirubin was 164 μmol/l. She was slightly lethargic but taking feeds reasonably.

a What is the probable cause of the jaundice?
b Name any special treatment that is likely to be required?
c What is the probable reason for her low birth weight?

CASE 10

A mother is worried that her 2½-year-old daughter does not talk.
The girl makes noises but no distinct words. She makes her needs
known by gesture. She is a healthy child. She can run and climb
stairs. She copies a circle with a pencil, and can build a tower of 8
cubes. She is dry by day, but wears nappies at night. She can
undress herself and eats with a spoon and fork.

She is the first child of parents who are both teachers, though
the mother has not gone out to work since the daughter arrived.
The pregnancy and perinatal history were normal.

a Should the mother be reassured that her daughter is essentially
   normal?
b What is the likely reason for the speech problem?
c What further investigation is required?

CASE 11

A 5-year-old boy develops pain in the right knee and the right
hand. He is not feverish and does not feel ill. Three days later a
purpuric rash becomes apparent, and is most prominent about the
ankles. His blood picture shows: Hb 13 g/dl; WBC $8.2 \times 10^9/l$;
platelets $180 \times 10^9/l$. There is no family history of a bleeding
disorder or similar rash. Apart from occasional 'wheezy bronchitis'
he has been well. He has had no immunisation because the mother
'does not believe in them'.

a What is the probable diagnosis?
b Name two additional symptoms and signs which may develop
   during the following weeks.
c What is the chest X-ray likely to show?

CASE 12

A 4-month-old infant presents with poor weight gain. He has always been a slow feeder, and in particular would only take small quantities of milk at a time. He has been a restless irritable baby who sweated a lot.

On examination his length is 62 cm and weight 4.8 kg. He looks pale. The pulse rate is 190/min, the respiratory rate 54/min. The blood pressure is 80/40. There is a grade 4/6 pansystolic murmur heard best to the left of the sternum. The liver is palpable 4 cm below the right costal margin. The pregnancy was complicated by severe vomiting in the first 3 months and a threatened miscarriage at 16 weeks. His birth weight was 3.1 kg.

a   What is the probable diagnosis?
b   Name two immediate (and simple) investigations which would help to establish a diagnosis.
c   Give three important therapeutic manoeuvres.

ANSWERS TO
MULTIPLE CHOICE QUESTIONS

Correct (True) responses are:

1. A B D E	22. A C	43. C D E
2. A B D E	23. A D E	44. B D
3. B D E	24. A C D E	45. A B C
4. B C D	25. A B C	46. A B C D
5. C D E	26. A C E	47. E
6. B C D	27. A B C D	48. A B D
7. A B C	28. B C D E	49. E
8. B C E	29. A B D E	50. A B C D
9. A C D E	30. B D	51. A
10. A B C	31. A B C D E	52. B C
11. B E	32. A D	53. A B
12. B C	33. A C	54. A B C E
13. B C D E	34. B C D	55. None
14. A C E	35. A B C D	56. C D E
15. C E	36. A B C D	57. B E
16. A B C D	37. A C D E	58. A B D E
17. B C D	38. A B C D E	59. A C D
18. A B C D E	39. B C E	60. B C D
19. C D E	40. A B E	61. A B C
20. B C	41. B C D	62. C E
21. C D E	42. A E	63. A E

64. A E

65. A B D

66. C

67. C D E

68. B C D E

69. A C D E

70. D E

71. B D

72. B C

73. A B C E

74. B C E

75. A B E

76. A D

77. C E

78. B D

79. A B C E

80. A B D

81. A B C E

82. A

83. A D

84. B C D

85. A B C E

86. C D E

87. C

88. C D E

89. C E

90. A B E

91. A C D E

92. A B D

93. A B D E

94. A C

95. C E

96. A B C

97. A B C E

98. A B

99. A B C

100. D

101. A B C

102. E

103. B C

104. A B D

105. B C D

106. A B D E

107. A B C E

108. B C D

109. A C E

110. B C D

111. A B C E

112. A B C D E

113. A C D

114. C

115. A C

116. None

117. A C E

118. B C

119. A E

120. A B E

121. B D E

122. A B E

123. None

124. B C E

125. C D E

126. None

127. C

128. A B C D

129. A C D

130. A C D E

131. B C E

132. A B C D

133. B C D

134. C

135. B C D E

136. A B D

137. A C D

138. B D

139. A B C D	152. B C D	165. A C D E
140. B D	153. A C	166. A C E
141. A B	154. A	167. A C D
142. A B C E	155. B C	168. A C E
143. A B E	156. D E	169. A B E
144. A B C D	157. A B E	170. C D
145. B C D	158. A B C D	171. B
146. A B C D	159. None	172. B C D
147. A D	160. A B	173. C D E
148. B C D E	161. B	174. A D E
149. A B D E	162. A B C D E	175. B C E
150. A C D E	163. None	
151. A B E	164. A B D E	

ANSWERS TO
CASE STUDIES

CASE 1

a   Rehydration with intravenous fluids. He is dehydrated and the vomiting suggests that he may not tolerate oral fluids.
b   A test feed during which the abdomen is palpated for a pyloric lump (i.e. pyloric stenosis).
c   Reassure the parents that umbilical herniae are common and harmless and that his will go by the age of 12 months.

CASE 2

a   Breath-holding attacks.
b   The child being hurt, angry or frustrated.
c   Excellent, she will 'grow out of them' by the age of 5.
d   No.

CASE 3

a   i. Salaam attack (infantile spasms).
    ii. A normal startle response in a normal baby.
b   Electroencephalograph. Infantile spasms are associated with hypsarrhythmia.
c   Most infants who have infantile spasms grow up to have recurrent seizures or mental handicap (or both of these).

CASE 4

a Idiopathic nephrotic syndrome.
b i. Serum albumin, which will be low.
    ii. Urine protein, which will be excessive.
c Troublesome, with recurrent attacks in childhood. Eventual cure and normal adult life are likely.
d Prednisone (or other corticosteroid).

CASE 5

a i. Acute asthma.
    ii. Lower respiratory tract infection, e.g. pneumonia.
b The presence in close relatives of:
    i. Similar attacks.
    ii. Hay fever, eczema or sensitivity rashes, i.e. 'atopy'.
c i. The 'runny nose' could be a sign of infection or allergic rhinitis (hay fever) either of which could lead to an attack of wheezing.
    ii. The 'holiday house' could bring him into contact with particular allergens, e.g. pollens in the appropriate season or, more likely, house dust mite which is notorious for nestling in unfrequented holiday cottages.
    iii. The 'birthday party' could cause him to have excessive excitement or exercise, either of which might bring on wheezing.
    iv. Allergy to haggis and the sound of bagpipes is a good idea, but in this case cannot be allowed.

CASE 6

a Herpetic stomatitis (hepatic gingivo-stomatitis).
b Primary infection with *herpesvirus hominis* (herpes simplex virus).
c It will not recur in the severe form; subsequent reactivation will cause merely a 'cold sore' on the lip.

CASE 7

a Iron deficiency (microcytic, hypochromic).
b Insufficient iron in diet because of feeding difficulty, and slowness to chew solids because of mental handicap.
c The perinatal history, because adverse events *in utero*, at birth, and in the neonatal period are particularly likely to cause brain damage.
d Cypriots are prone to glucose-6-phosphate dehydrogenase deficiency and to thalassaemia major, either of which is associated with splenomegaly.

CASE 8

a *Staphylococcus pyogenes*. Tuberculosis is also possible.
b Cystic fibrosis
 i. Offensive loose faeces.
 ii. Sweat sodium and chloride measurement.
 iii. Analysis of faeces.
 iv. Analysis of duodenal juice.

CASE 9

a Physiological jaundice (immaturity of the liver enzyme glucuronyl transferrase).
b None is likely to be required though, if the rate of rise of bilirubin became excessive, phenobarbitone or blue light phototherapy could be helpful.
c A racial or familial characteristic.

CASE 10

a No. The girl is normal or advanced in all phases of development except speech or language and a reason should be sought.

b Deafness. The home circumstances make it likely that the child is being exposed to plenty of language from her mother; therefore it is probable that she can not hear it. In a poor home, with a disinterested uncommunicative or absent mother, lack of exposure to language would need to be excluded.

c Hearing tests and examination of the ears.

CASE 11

a Henoch–Schönlein syndrome.

b i. Abdominal pain (also diarrhoea and vomiting).

ii. Haematuria with or without proteinuria. (Henoch first reported the occurrence of nephritis in this syndrome when he was over the age of 90; there is hope for some of us yet).

c A normal appearance.

CASE 12

a Cardiac failure secondary to a congenital heart lesion (probably a ventricular septal defect).

b i. Chest X-ray.

ii. ECG.

c i. Oxygen.

ii. Diuretic.

iii. Digitalisation.

iv. Tube-feeding.